Ready, Set, Radiation

How to Prepare for Radiation Therapy Treatments

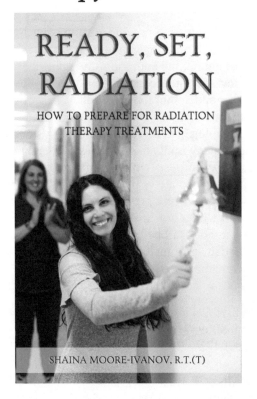

READY, SET,
RADIATION

HOW TO PREPARE FOR RADIATION
THERAPY TREATMENTS

SHAINA MOORE-IVANOV, R.T.(T)

By Shaina Moore-Ivanov, R.T.(T)

Copyright

ISBN:
Paperback: 979-8-9909471-0-8
Hardcover: 979-8-9909471-1-5
Ebook: 979-8-9909471-2-2

Book Cover by Alisa Charnley
Edited by Diane Timmons and Heather Moore

Ornamentation designed by Freepik.com

First edition 2024

Printed in the United States of America

Thank You and Dedication

I would like to send a special thank you to the healthcare workers taking care of patients affected by cancer. Oncology is a special field that takes a special person to do their job well. Thank you for stepping up to make a difference.

I would like to dedicate this book to all cancer warriors, past and present, and their support systems. Cancer sucks, and I am so sorry that you are going through this! You are more than your diagnosis, and you are not alone.

In Remembrance

In loving memory of my dad, Darrell Edward Moore, who lost his battle with cancer. We miss you.

Purpose

Cancer is one of the scariest words to hear in any language. Understanding cancer and deciding how to combat it is a tough and personal decision to make, and it is also an incredibly vulnerable experience for anyone to have to go through. No one should enter this chapter of their lives without the tools they will need to walk through this journey confidently and fearlessly.

I wrote this book for that reason: to equip patients everywhere with the knowledge they will need to navigate radiation therapy treatments. My goal is to help every patient walking through the front door of any radiation oncology department to feel fully prepared and confident that they understand and know exactly what they are getting themselves into. There is so much information out there, but there are so few resources that organize that information in a digestible way. I hope this book helps with that by offering at least one resource to help make this chapter of your life more understandable and less overwhelming.

Good luck to you on your cancer journey! You've got this!

Table of Contents

Disclaimer

This is a general disclaimer that I am <u>not</u> a licensed physician. Rather, I am a radiation therapist who has spent over three years treating patients in the radiation oncology setting. Over this time, I have also had the privilege to join so many patients in their fight against cancer. I am simply sharing the knowledge gained through my own experiences throughout my career.

Everything in this book is meant strictly for supplemental guidance purposes only and is not meant to take the place of medical advice. ***Please consult a physician regarding your specific situation and healthcare needs!***

Introduction

When most people think about cancer treatment, they think of "chemotherapy." However, there are so many different routes other than chemotherapy that a person's cancer treatment journey might follow. Some other options may include surgery, immunotherapy, or homeopathic approaches. Some people even choose to not pursue treatment at all. However, radiation therapy is a big one that most people don't even *know* about until they know someone undergoing treatment or are about to get treatments themselves. Heck—my dad had cancer and I didn't even know what radiation therapy was until over 10 years later!

I am now a practicing radiation therapist who treats patients battling cancer daily. This is the reason I am writing this book. Every day, I see new patients walk in for their first appointment looking terrified and overwhelmed with anxiety because they have no idea what to expect. There is such a scarcity of organized guidance available for patients expecting to begin treatments. I cannot imagine how scary it must be to get the news that you have cancer. Or, even more so, how incredibly terrifying it would be to agree to undergo a course of treatment that I know absolutely nothing about and for which I cannot prepare myself.

The goal of this book is to introduce you and your support system to radiation treatment as it pertains to cancer. There is so much to learn about in the field of radiation therapy, but I do not wish to overwhelm you by repeating a ton of scientific and medical jargon that will not benefit you in any way. Instead, I hope to guide you through this treatment journey, explaining as much as **necessary** along the way with a personable approach. In doing this, I hope to help you get through radiation treatments to that final day where you can ring the celebratory bell so loud and hard that you will never doubt your capability and strength ever again.

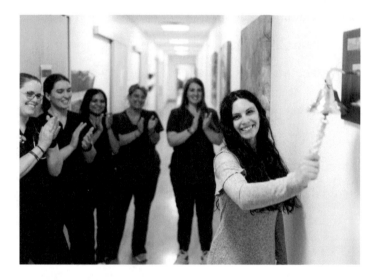

Figure 1 A patient celebrates her final radiation treatment by ringing the bell. Patients have the choice of ringing the bell on their last day. The bell does not indicate that they are cancer-free, but that they have accomplished this milestone of their journey. Image courtesy of Red Fox Photography.

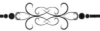

CHAPTER 1
Cancer Diagnosis—
What Comes Next?

The time following a cancer diagnosis is such a whirlwind. You are still trying to process the news, and now you must decide what to do next, too. First off, I am so sorry this is happening to you! Cancer truly sucks! Unfortunately, this will feel like a very scary time for you and your family, and I cannot tell you this journey will be easy. Take a moment to let the swarm of information sink in because this can all become overwhelming very quickly. Try to begin to process everything so when you are ready to think about the next step, you can do so rationally and clearly.

My biggest piece of advice to anyone is to advocate for yourself and to ask questions! Ask questions no matter how silly you think they might be, and certainly even if you think it is a "dumb" question. People always say there are "no dumb questions," but this is especially true when they are concerning your health. For your peace of mind, ask questions at every step of the way! Ask every question that you can think of to your nurse, your therapists, and your doctors to gather as much information as possible so when the time comes to make the decision, you can do so feeling educated and armed with the knowledge of what you are about to walk into. While I encourage you to utilize this book as a starting point to help you gather information, you must get clarification from your physician regarding any areas of concern you may have. Every treatment center is different, so procedures and processes will certainly vary from clinic to clinic.

I also suggest you surround yourself with people you trust to help you make important healthcare decisions. Your treatment plan options will be determined by many different factors including your diagnosis, prognosis, age, and comorbidities. Your team of trained healthcare professionals will assemble a list of treatment options for you. They will use their abundant research, data, and knowledge to determine what those options are, and they will make their best recommendations based on what they know, what they have seen, and the research available to them surrounding your specific diagnosis.

Many different treatment options might be recommended to you on your cancer journey. Surgery, chemotherapy, radiation therapy, immunotherapy, and clinical trials are the typical options that most patients will learn about. It may be recommended that you undergo treatment utilizing one of these modalities on its own, a couple of them together, or you may even find that you'll undergo each of these treatments at some point throughout your journey.

One important concept to take note of is that not all types of cancer or tumors respond well to radiation. The same goes for chemotherapy. Surgery is also not possible in every circumstance, as a tumor may be wrapped around important vessels or be too close to critical structures. The reason I share this information is to explain why one or many of these options might not be an option for you and your cancer diagnosis specifically. Again, I encourage you to speak to your licensed healthcare provider to explain your options in depth.

If you feel like you need or want a second opinion, get one! This is your life, your body, and your peace of mind! Your team will respect your decision and understand that you are not condemning their ability. Get your second opinion, if that is what you want, and give yourself a little peace of mind! The treatment you choose to get is entirely up to you, and it is important that you feel confident in that choice. With that being said, you need to be aware of how urgent it is for you to begin your treatment so you can be swift in getting that second opinion if needed. This is a great discussion to have with your medical and/or radiation oncologist.

CHAPTER 2
What is Radiation Therapy?

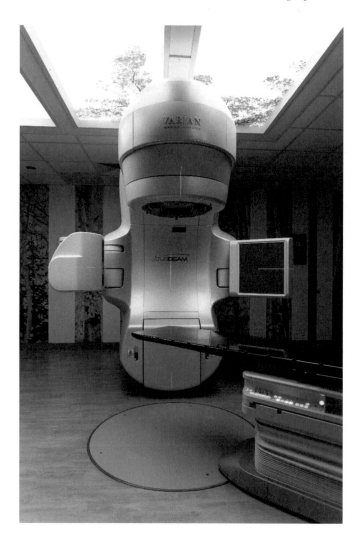

Figure 2 Varian TrueBeam Linear Accelerator. Image courtesy of Red Fox Photography.

As you might recall from some foggy high school biology class note-taking, the human body is comprised of cells. Cells contain DNA, the hereditary material in humans. This hereditary material is the most sensitive part of the cell and is located within the nucleus.

Radiation therapy is a type of cancer treatment that utilizes high-energy beams of particles to kill DNA. Killing DNA causes cells to die and tumors to shrink. It is important to note that while we are targeting unhealthy cells, it is inevitable that some healthy tissue will be damaged, as well. Rest assured that your team will create your treatment plan to minimize the healthy tissue that is receiving treatment. Cancer cells are not able to recover from the radiation treatments, while your healthy cells are indeed able to regenerate and recover over time.

Different types of particles are used in radiation therapy treatments. Of these, the most commonly used are electrons, photons, and protons. Patients being treated on a linear accelerator (LINAC) most often are treated utilizing photons. In layman's terms, the LINAC essentially has a sequence in place that accelerates a beam of electrons into a tungsten target which creates photons. Adjusting the speed at which the electrons are accelerated produces different energies of photons. These different energy levels help the radiation oncology team determine how deep into a person's body the radiation can be delivered.

Different types of radiation treatments include external beam radiation therapy and internal radiation therapy (brachytherapy). The type of therapy that you will receive will depend on many factors and will ultimately be recommended directly by your physician. You may even receive multiple types of radiation and particle beams depending on your treatment plan. The most common type of treatment is external beam radiation therapy utilizing electrons and photons. For this reason, this is the type of treatment that this book will focus on, although I will briefly summarize other types of treatments.

One technique used in external beam radiation to ensure the conformal treatment to the area of focus is the use of multileaf collimators or MLCs. MLCs are motorized metallic leaves that essentially shape the treatment beam as it exits the machine (as shown below).

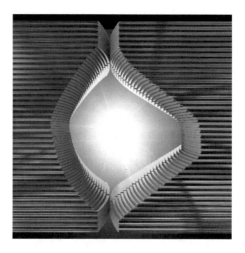

Figure 3 MultiLeaf Collimator. MLCs help to shape the treatment beam as it exits the treatment machine. Image(s) courtesy of Elekta.

Some things that might factor into your physician's recommendation for your treatments include, but are not limited to, the following:

What is your diagnosis?

Meaning, what type of cancer do you have? At what stage or grade is it? What types of treatment does your specific cancer type respond well to and which treatment has research to support this?

What is your prognosis?

What is the likely outcome of this disease? It is determined by asking what the extent of the cancer is. Was it caught early and localized, or has it already metastasized (or spread) elsewhere in your body? What is your life expectancy with or without treatment? Can you be cured?

Typically, early detection is our best bet against fighting cancer. If the cancer was discovered early enough that it has not yet spread, you will often have a better prognosis and therefore a higher chance of being "cured." Sadly, metastatic disease and high-grade tumors pose a more serious threat to your body and result in a poorer prognosis. Your team of medical professionals will take all of this (and much more) into account before making a recommendation for treatment.

What is the goal of treatment?

Speak to your radiation oncologist about the intent of the treatment that you might pursue to better decide what is best for you. Radiation therapy can be used both curatively and in palliative cases. Curative therapy is as the name suggests and has the goal of "curing" the patient's disease. Patients receiving curative doses of radiation might receive a greater number of treatments than patients receiving palliative care. However, sometimes a patient might receive a "curative dose" without the intent of being able to cure the disease. This curative dose may, however, serve to increase a person's quality of life as well as help to prolong their life expectancy.

Palliative care aims to treat patient's symptoms to help increase their quality of life. (Palliative Care in Musculoskeletal Oncology - PMC (nih.gov). Palliative care is quite common with patients who have bone metastases. Bone metastases can be very painful as the cancer is "eating" at the bone. Radiation can be an incredible means to shrink these metastatic lesions, slow down tumor growth, and relieve cancer-related symptoms like pain or bleeding.

How deep or superficial is the treatment site?

The different types of particles can penetrate to different depths, based on the characteristics of the different particles. A physician might choose to treat a patient using electrons if they are trying to treat more superficially located areas, often less than a few centimeters in depth. Because they do not travel very far into the body, they are most often used to treat cancers on the skin or near the body's surface. Breast scar sterilization can be achieved with electrons. We will also use electron therapy to treat keloids after they have been surgically removed to prevent them from recurring. While electron treatment can be used in other cases, these are simply the most common uses that I have seen while working as a radiation therapist.

As explained previously, the different types of particles and energies have specific characteristics in terms of the depth to which they can penetrate a person's body. Photons penetrate deeper than electrons typically would, which is why electrons are often used to treat more superficial lesions. Therefore, one characteristic of electron beams is that they decrease skin sparing, meaning that your skin will receive a higher dose than it would using a different type of energy. Electron treatments may be conducted utilizing a linear accelerator. Some dermatology clinics use particle accelerators. (American Cancer Society, Getting external beam radiation therapy). The electron beams are invisible and cannot be felt while receiving treatment. [i]

Photons or X-rays are the most commonly utilized type of radiation in most cancer centers. Like electrons, photon beams cannot be felt as they pass through the patient's body to reach the targeted cells. Photon beams have higher energy levels and therefore can penetrate deeper into the body. Because of this, however, they can damage healthy cells on the way to and after reaching the cancerous cells. There are many different techniques your physician's team can utilize to decrease and minimize the dose to healthy tissue while targeting unhealthy tissue.

How Healthy are You?

As with medications, it is important for the physician to know your other comorbidities to help them determine if radiation is a practical and safe treatment option for you. Can your body handle the treatment? Someone who is not physically stable may not be a great candidate for radiation until they are a little bit better, for example. Please speak to your medical provider to determine what type of radiation treatment, if any, might be best in your specific set of circumstances.

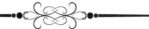

CHAPTER 3
Demystifying a Common Misconception

B efore we go any further, I would like to quickly clarify that radiation treatment is not only used to treat people who have cancer. While this is undoubtedly its primary and most common use, there are a few other radiation therapy applications in healthcare. While this is not an exhaustive list, radiation therapy can also be used for the following:

Keloids: Radiation therapy can treat the scar following the surgical removal of keloids to help prevent their recurrence. This is often done within 24 hours of the surgical removal of keloids.

Transplants: Radiation therapy can help prepare a person's body for a stem cell or bone marrow transplant. While this can sometimes be done on patients with leukemia, it is not always the case. This type of treatment will be covered more in-depth in a later section of this book, "Total Body Irradiation."

Heterotopic Bone Ossification: Heterotopic ossification is mature, and lamellar bone formation is in soft tissues where bone does not usually exist. It is commonly seen following trauma or surgical intervention of periarticular soft tissue. Radiation therapy can be used to prevent heterotopic bone growth following trauma, surgery, or hip/knee replacement.[ii]

Dupuytren's Contracture: Patients suffering from Dupuytren's Contracture might present with nodules in the tendons in their hands. Radiation treatments, while not extremely common in the United States, can be used in the early stages to help soften the nodules and prevent contractions from occurring. [iii]

Inflammatory Conditions: Some clinics have begun using radiation to treat inflammatory conditions like plantar fasciitis, tendonitis, and osteoarthritis.

Benign Skin Conditions: Less commonly, some clinics also use radiation to treat conditions like warts and psoriasis.

Superior Vena Cava Syndrome (SVCS): SVCS is caused by the occlusion or obstruction of the superior vena cava and can be life-threatening when the airway becomes obstructed. Radiation therapy has proven to be very effective in relieving airway obstruction and reducing symptoms associated with SVCS.

Spinal Cord Compression: Radiation therapy is also used in palliative cases to treat spinal cord compressions (resulting from cancer metastasizing to the spine) and in cases of uncontrolled tumor hemorrhaging to prevent too much blood loss. [iv]

CHAPTER 4

Radiation Therapy Treatment Facility Types

One of the first and possibly most essential questions to ask yourself at the beginning of this journey is where you should go to receive your treatments. Location is significant and could become a limiting factor for you. If you want to be treated in a different state or country, you must think about the financial implications of that decision.

While I have seen patients travel across the country to be seen by whom they felt was "the best team in the country," it is essential to understand that your medical insurance may or may not cover treatment conducted out of state. Call your insurance company to figure that out. In my experience, patients coming to the United States from another country often would pay out of pocket for their treatments. However, you should still talk to your insurance company to determine your eligibility if that is an option you wish to consider! Larger hospitals or teaching facilities might offer some humanitarian efforts where the cost of treatment could be subsidized or covered for patients without insurance. Please do your research and have all the information confirmed by someone from the facility before you go in to avoid any surprises or delays in treatment.

Within the United States, different insurance companies may allow you different options for where you can receive your treatments. It is very important to learn and review your options before deciding on where to go. While all physicians will do their best to optimize your treatment, there are many other factors that are more practical and could be worth considering.

More extensive facilities such as hospitals are excellent because you have almost everything you need under one roof. These might include MRIs, CT scans, blood draws, CT simulators specifically for radiation oncology, emergency rooms, medical oncology with chemotherapy centers, pharmacies, or anything else you would need during your cancer journey. The convenience of attending all possible appointments in the same location is understandably essential to some patients.

On the other hand, many larger hospitals are located in large cities. Large cities often have extra traffic, confusing or stressful parking, parking costs, or higher patient volumes. However, public transportation is much more available in these locations. This could be a great option if you rely on public transportation to get to your appointments!

Another great thing about larger, big-name facilities is that they are more likely to offer alternative methods of care. Many smaller clinics are not equipped to treat rare diagnoses, so you may be referred to a larger hospital with physicians who specialize in or are more familiar with your diagnosis. Some clinics may not accept pediatric patients and will refer them to children's centers with physicians specializing in treating children. Also, different types of treatment machines will vary from clinic to clinic. Some machines are more specialized and can treat patients using different techniques. You may have heard or seen advertisements on the radio or TV about "proton therapy." There are not as many proton centers in the country as there are traditional therapy clinics, so this could limit your options if you are determined to receive proton therapy.

Make sure to talk to your physician about other affiliated clinical sites attached to the hospital you are interested in. Many larger radiation oncology departments have physicians who practice out of more than one location in their network. Be sure to ask your doctor if there are other options for the location of your treatment and be open and honest about where the most convenient location for you would be.

Smaller facilities and cancer centers can also be excellent in many ways. Parking might be more convenient and is often free, mainly if the clinic is in a smaller city or suburb. The buildings are often smaller, so you might experience less anxiety about getting lost. Lastly, because they don't come with the city's traffic, traveling to and from treatment might also be a little more convenient. This would be especially helpful for someone who might have to continue working for the duration of their treatments, as you'd be able to zip right in and back out fairly quickly.

If you got nothing else from this section, I hope you feel empowered to choose a treatment location, knowing there are plenty of ways to filter your decision. This is **YOUR** treatment! Know your options and decide what works best for YOU. Insurance can undoubtedly play a huge factor in which facilities you can go to, but it is always worth it to weigh your options and make an informed decision.

CHAPTER 5
Factors to Consider When Deciding Where to Undergo Treatment

How far will I be driving each day to and from treatment? How long is my commute?

Keep in mind that one common side effect of radiation treatments is fatigue. Anxiety or pain medications, as well as a plethora of other drugs, tend to cause drowsiness in some people. If you are driving yourself, I beg you to please choose a clinic that you can make it to and from *safely*.

Is my diagnosis rare?

Some larger clinics may have been more exposed to rare diagnoses than smaller clinics. Therefore, they might have better insight into the best techniques to treat your specific diagnosis.

How many treatment machines does the clinic have?

Linear accelerators are pieces of equipment that utilize advanced technology and software. They are expensive and highly sophisticated but are not infallible to faults and broken parts. When a treatment machine is not functioning correctly, larger clinics might be able to get you treated on a different but compatible machine so that you will not have to miss a day of treatment. Smaller clinics with only one linear accelerator cannot do that. Fortunately, the engineers working on these machines are capable of getting the machine back up and running pretty quickly. It does not happen very often that a machine needs repair, so this is not something you should be highly concerned about or to base your decision solely on. I merely mention this as a tiny thing to keep in mind since it can occur.

Does the clinic have a good reputation?

Read the reviews online about the oncology department. They can be very insightful! Also, ask if anyone you know has been treated there and what their experience was like. In healthcare, we strive to create a caring environment for all. Unfortunately, some clinics fall short of that goal for various reasons.

From the bottom of my heart, wherever you choose to go, I genuinely hope you find the care you deserve! Please let someone know if you get to a clinic and feel you're not being treated kindly and respectfully. I sincerely doubt the person with whom you had a bad interaction intentionally was rude. Let someone know because we, too, are humans who have bad days and need to take a short break and be reminded to put our game face on!

What appointment times are available at each clinical site?

Many clinics operate within the general business hours of 7 a.m.- 5 p.m. Some might treat later into the evenings, while others open earlier and close earlier. Be sure to ask about this upfront if you are concerned.

Can I choose my treatment times, or is it based on a schedule?

Radiation Oncology is very different from other areas of the hospital, especially in the way we schedule patients for their daily treatment appointments. Some clinics may not be able to guarantee you a specific appointment time until the first day of treatment. Others might be able to schedule you out within a couple of days before your first treatment. Unfortunately, this is a variable practice that is different from clinic to clinic. Still, I will say that it is very common for patients to be scheduled for their remaining treatments at the time of their first treatment appointment.

We know this can be very inconvenient for scheduling other necessary medical appointments or coordinating rides to treatment. We also know that it is hard to plan your life around the treatments rather than plan the treatments around your life. The problem is that we have new patients starting or completing *their* treatments daily. Sometimes, patients will be scheduled to complete treatment, but they might be sick and miss a day, which pushes their treatment schedule back a day. A patient might experience complications outside of treatment that cause them to be delayed by a few days. The doctor can also decide that the patient needs a few additional treatments. These are just a few examples of situations that might arise on any given day that impact scheduling.

Anything has the potential to change the treatment machine's schedule from day to day, so we do not know what times we will have available until we are very close to your first scheduled appointment. While we truly do realize that this is very frustrating, we ask for your patience, understanding, and flexibility. Treatment plans typically range anywhere from one to eight weeks in total, so it's for a short period that we are asking for this flexibility and offer you the encouragement that you will get through these treatments and back to your normal routine shortly!

If the specific time for your daily treatments is something causing you anxiety, please let your therapists know at the time of your CT simulation appointment so they can make a note in your chart as to your preference for treatment **timeframe.** While a *specific* time can't be guaranteed, we can certainly *do our best* to get you into a *timeframe* that might work for you. Again, we do ask for a little flexibility as we have new patients beginning treatment each day and so our schedules are constantly changing.

Please also try to keep in mind that there are so many other patients already receiving treatments and that we are trying to get everyone started on their treatment courses as soon as possible. If the times you are offered are not convenient, you are more than welcome to ask to be put on a waitlist for a more convenient time. Being inflexible with treatment times is not going to serve you well when a clinic simply has no other appointment times to offer you.

We understand that you have important things going on in your life, and we do not want you to miss them, but many other patients also need to be scheduled. We will try our best to accommodate you, but sometimes requests can only be made possible by being put on a waitlist for the time you want. We do not wish to start on the wrong foot with our patients being upset with us over treatment times, especially when that is something that is out of even *our* control. We do apologize for any inconveniences in advance and truly do strive to make things as easy and seamless as possible while we are caring for you.

Will you be treated like a person or like a number?

This one is not dependent on the size of the clinic, although it is certainly easier for smaller clinics with lower patient volume to give you more of their time each day. All clinics and medical teams should treat you professionally and with respect, but please remember that many other patients are scheduled for treatment, too. Clinics must focus on staying on schedule and getting you in and out of the door so that they don't take the next patient in late.

Depending on the staff, some clinics will offer a more personal approach and get to know you throughout your treatment. If I were to undergo something as delicate and emotional as cancer treatment, I'd certainly like to be treated as a whole person rather than as an appointment time. It can be hard to gauge the atmosphere simply from a consult with your physician, but this is where it is so crucial to get recommendations from family, friends, and Google reviews if a personal approach is something important to you. Some patients prefer to just get their treatment and not converse, and that is okay, too. We can usually figure out when patients want to skip the small talk and try to respect their cues.

What is the turnaround time from consultation with your radiation oncologist to your first treatment day?

This is a great question to ask your physician on the day of your consultation! Most people with a cancer diagnosis want to begin treatment right away for obvious reasons. Radiation therapy is a prescribed treatment course; it is not as simple as filling a prescription bottle and slapping a sticker on it with your name so you can pick it up at the pharmacy (not that filling a prescription at a pharmacy is necessarily a simple task either, FYI).

There is a whole team of medical professionals who take part in your treatment journey that most people never know about because you will never meet them. Planning your treatment can be a very lengthy process and the time it takes will depend on how busy the clinic is, how complicated your treatment might be, the area you are treating, the technique your physician is planning to use, and so much more.

Keep in mind that many other patients are also waiting to start their treatments. At busy clinics, one patient might have to complete treatment before another can begin theirs, simply due to the lack of appointment slots available. Wait times can be up to a month for certain locations! Others might be as quick as a couple of days! It all depends. This is a conversation to have with your doctor when you decide where you would like to get treatment.

What are the costs associated with treatment?

I'm sure you know by now that the cost of anything healthcare-related is not readily available with a simple Google search. Finding all the costs associated with treatment can be tricky, but it isn't impossible. The best thing you can do would be to call your insurance company and request all of that information from them. If you know where you might be getting treatment, how many treatments you need, and the type of technique your radiation oncologist plans to use, you can get a pretty good estimate of the out-of-pocket costs. Coinsurance, deductibles, facility fees, medications you know you'll need, etc., are some of the costs you should be inquiring about.

Keep in mind that there might be other costs that aren't strictly insurance-based. Creams and wound dressings might be recommended to you. Sometimes these items are not covered by insurance, which is something to keep in mind. Larger facilities may charge parking fees. Some clinics can validate your parking pass to provide you with free parking, but other clinics cannot. If you do not have a vehicle, there may be transportation costs to get you to or from your treatment.

Pro tip: some insurance companies cover shared transportation to medical appointments, so it could be worth looking into.

Lastly, many patients can continue working throughout their treatment. Others, physically or emotionally, cannot. While this truly depends on the individual, it is something that only YOU will know. Fatigue is a very common side effect of treatment, so knowing yourself and whether or not you'll need to take time off of work to complete treatments and get better is important. Talk to your Human Resources department at work to learn more about FMLA and other policies that can help you decide if taking time off work is possible and plausible for you and your situation.

What other resources can the facility offer you?

Many cancer treatment facilities offer a variety of additional resources. Some may offer the resources of social workers, nutritionists, and financial help including housing, transportation assistance, or parking cost assistance. Some clinics offer free parking, while others do not. If anything is causing you concern that might act as a roadblock to your receiving treatment, please share your concerns with your doctor at your consultation to see if there are ways the clinic can assist you. Remember that at the end of the day, cancer centers are businesses that are competing to earn your "business." Make sure you're doing your research to get the best treatment, customer service, and *care* that you are not only *paying* for but that you *deserve*.

CHAPTER 6
Consultation with a Radiation Oncologist

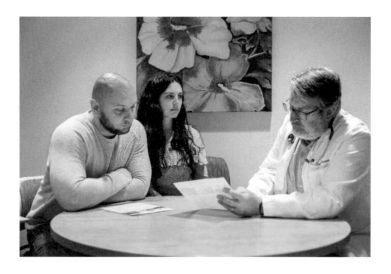

Figure 4 A prospective patient attends a consultation with a radiation oncologist. Here, she will learn all about what to expect and the next steps. It can be very helpful to bring someone with you to help understand and ask questions. Image courtesy of Red Fox Photography.

After you have met with your medical team to go over your diagnosis and treatment options, you might have learned that radiation is an option for you. Next, you will need to schedule a consultation appointment with a radiation oncologist. When you go in for this appointment, try to have your list of questions ready for the physician. They will explain the treatment process to you and review information about your specific type of cancer. They will go over different radiation treatment options, goals and expected results of treatment, and any possible side effects that you might expect as a result of the treatments. They may also ask you to sign a patient treatment consent form.

After you have agreed to undergo treatment, someone from your chosen clinic's staff will call you or reach out to you to schedule your "CT simulation" appointment. This is your next step. The person who reaches out to set up your simulation appointment should explain any important steps that you need to take to prepare for your simulation. If they don't, use the online patient portal where your appointment can be visualized and check to see if there are any instructions attached to the appointment. Different treatment areas might require different preparation steps, and some areas simply require no preparation at all. Some treatment facilities do not require preparation steps in general. Simply follow the instructions you are given, and everything should be just fine for your first day in radiation oncology!

CHAPTER 7
Preparing for Your CT-Simulation

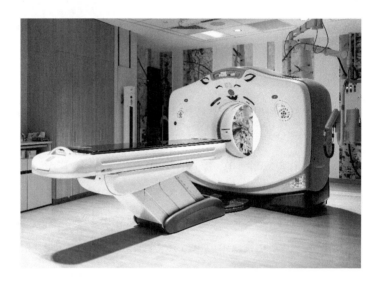

Figure 5 The photo above depicts a CT-Simulator, a medical imaging device utilized in the Radiation Oncology department. CT scans are performed to aid the physician and the planning team in developing a treatment plan. Image courtesy of Red Fox Photography.

While this might vary from clinic to clinic, some **typical** preparation steps are as follows for these different regions of the body:

- **Prostate**: Please arrive with a full bladder and empty rectum. Sometimes the patient may be asked to complete a fleet enema for their CT Simulation to ensure an empty rectum. The patient may instead be asked to simply have a bowel movement before being scanned. These instructions will be asked of you for the duration of your full course of treatment.

- **Liver/Stomach/Pancreas**: Patients receiving treatment to the abdominal area may be asked to follow "nothing by mouth" (NPO) instructions. This is asking the patient not to eat or drink anything for a certain length of time before their scan. This will likely be asked of you for the duration of your full course of treatment if it is asked of you for the simulation. If you take medications at a specific time of the day and think this might affect that schedule, let your physician know. Often, taking your medications with a sip of water while NPO is still okay. **Do not follow NPO instructions unless they are ordered directly by your physician!** Doing so could be dangerous if you are not medically cleared to safely do so!

- **Bladder**: Patients receiving treatments to the bladder might be asked to have an empty bladder for both the simulation and each daily treatment appointment. This means using the bathroom (urinating) as closely as possible to your appointment time to achieve an empty bladder. Not drinking water for a short period before your scan would help facilitate this, but follow the specific instructions given to you by your physician or nurse.

- **Brain, Head, and Neck:** Patients being treated to the brain, head, or neck areas will likely be prescribed treatments utilizing a mask. The masks used for treatment essentially clip down to the treatment table, immobilizing the patient. Patients who struggle with claustrophobia might need to consider anxiety medication. **Please consult with your radiation oncology physician if you are claustrophobic to receive their medical opinion as to whether anxiety medication is right for you.**

CHAPTER 8
CT Simulation – general information

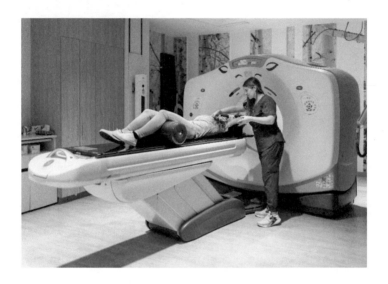

Figure 6 The radiation therapist is getting the patient into an ideal treatment position at the time of the simulation. Image courtesy of Red Fox Photography.

Your first appointment in radiation oncology after your consultation is complete will likely be for CT Simulation. It is highly recommended that you wear comfortable clothing that can be easily removed as you may need to change into a gown. Be sure to have followed all preparation instructions, if there were any, and please plan to arrive at least 15 minutes early. Some clinics are extremely busy, so if you arrive late you may need to reschedule your appointment. Arriving early will give you extra time to figure out the parking situation, get yourself to the correct building, get checked in, to fill out any paperwork that might still be needed, for staff to review or explain what is expected of you for the day, or to allow yourself extra time to ask any questions that you still have.

The purpose of the CT simulation appointment is for the treatment team to decide on the best position for you to be in while you receive your radiation treatments. The team is "simulating" the position that you will be in for treatment, hence, the name CT simulation. This appointment also allows the team to obtain the CT imaging that will then be utilized to plan your treatments.

At most clinics, radiation therapists are the medical professionals who complete your CT simulation. They will get you set up in the correct position that your doctor has in mind for you, and the therapists will conduct the CT scan. There might be periods where it appears as though nothing is happening or like maybe they forgot about you. I promise that they did not! The therapist is simply waiting for the physician to review the scan and determine if they are happy with how the patient is set up on the table. Once the doctor has agreed that the scan and setup are ideal for creating a treatment plan, we can then mark your skin with the method that you previously agreed to.

To get you set up in the ideal treatment position, your radiation therapists will need to expose the treatment region. While we do our best to respect the modesty of patients, there may be times when the treatment area may need to remain uncovered for periods of time. This is necessary for a couple of different reasons. One reason is to help them determine where to begin the scan. There are protocols set in place at each facility that are very specific to the area of treatment. We do not scan your entire body because we aren't going to be *treating* your entire body. Remember that CT scans do give off small amounts of radiation, and our goal is to decrease unnecessary radiation exposure whenever possible. Another reason is that this appointment is also when your team will mark your skin to indicate to your treatment team where to begin each day. The skin must be uncovered for us to be able to make those markings.

The skin markings that I just mentioned are very important! I want to clarify this piece of information because it is the one piece of information that is often a shock to patients when they come in for their simulation appointment. Some clinics simply draw on the patient's skin with paint markers or permanent markers and place a waterproof sticker over them to preserve the marks. Other clinics believe that this method is not great because many patients will lose these stickers before their first treatment. To prevent this from happening, these clinics will give permanent skin markings called tattoos. When tattoos are given, the therapist will place a small amount of ink either directly on the skin or into the top of the needle and will then use the needle to deposit that ink just below the skin's surface.

Whichever way the clinic chooses to get this done, it is very important to follow the instructions given to you on preserving those marks. The biggest benefit to being given permanent tattoos is that you cannot lose them, and they will permanently indicate where you will receive treatment. Your treatment team will know without a doubt that this is where they need to align to each day for your treatment. If, for any reason, you need to be treated again someday, a trained eye will be able to detect these "tattoos" and will know where you have received treatment in the past.

Once the tattoos/skin markings are complete, you will be able to change back into your clothing, ask any final questions you may still have, and then be on your way. There are sometimes emergency cases that require simulation and treatment to be performed on the same day, but if you are not in critical condition, you will likely be scheduled to start your treatment on another day.

CHAPTER 9

Tattoos, Patient Autonomy, and Self-Advocacy

If you get nothing else from this section of the book, I hope you understand that getting tattooed is completely, unquestionably, 100% YOUR CHOICE. Some religions are totally against tattooing the body. Other people have been stuck with so many needles that they can't stand the idea of getting stuck with another. Some people have a phobia of needles. Even if you simply do not WANT them, you are allowed to say "no." You have complete autonomy over your healthcare decisions and will be required to sign a consent form indicating that you agree to receive tattoos.

Your physician might strongly encourage you to agree to tattoos. Please let your therapists know if you do not wish to receive tattoos and they will figure out another way to get the job done. Some clinics are working towards becoming tattoo-less centers. While tattoos aren't used at every single radiation treatment facility, they are still commonly practiced because they are helpful to the therapists when setting you up for treatment each day. For reference, they will be about the size of a freckle, and you probably won't even be able to tell they are there.

If you reject getting tattooed, the tattoos will likely be traded for the stickers that I previously mentioned. Be prepared to do your absolute best to keep those stickers on your body. This can be quite difficult to achieve depending on the area being marked, especially when the weather is warmer. Sweating in the breast and pelvic areas can make keeping those stickers on very tough to do. I have seen this become a very stressful matter for some of the patients I have treated, especially when it came to attending weddings or going to the beach or a pool on vacations. For these reasons, I highly recommend you take a moment to thoroughly think this through before you make your final decision. Now that we've thoroughly examined the art of tattooing in the radiation oncology department, let's review treatment positions.

Because cancer can be located anywhere in the body, and since each body shape is different, there is no "one-size-fits-all" treatment position for patients. This is the reason for the simulation. Your team will determine the best position for you and your specific treatment. There are some treatment positions that are more common for specific treatment sites which I will review.

Before I share these, I would like to encourage you to advocate for yourself during this appointment. Many patients are scheduled for radiation while they are still healing from surgeries or other procedures. Mobility of different areas of the body can be a limiting factor for the position that you may be required to be in for treatment. If bringing your arms up above your head is asked of you and it causes an immense amount of pain to shoot down your shoulder or causes your hands to go numb, we want to know these things! The simulation appointment will be much shorter than some of your days of treatment, so you must maintain this simulation position for the length of your daily treatments. You cannot move while in the required position receiving radiation treatments because we want to ensure that the correct body parts are receiving the correct amounts of radiation.

Once your simulation is complete, that is the position you will be expected to maintain throughout the course of your treatment, so I implore you to PLEASE be vocal at the time of your simulation about whether or not the position you are asked to lay in causes you a severe amount of discomfort. The team will try to do a little arts and crafts and a lot of finagling to get you into a treatment position that finds a balance between your comfort level and the position needed to get you treated properly.

Keep in mind that the setup positions I share are common positioning techniques, but it is possible that you may not be in these exact positions. Different hospitals and clinics treat their patients with different techniques and utilize different immobilization devices. The information I am about to share regarding CT simulation/treatment positions is strictly for guidance purposes. Please ask your physician if they have an idea of how you will be positioned if this is something causing you anxiety.

Depending on the clinic, you may be given your first treatment appointment time at the end of your simulation, or you may be told that you will receive a call soon to get that appointment scheduled. Please try to be patient! Busier or larger clinics might have longer wait times to be able to begin your treatments than a smaller clinic. It depends on the current patient load, the urgency to begin, and how many patients simulated before you and are still waiting to begin their treatments.

As I mentioned before, your CT scan from your simulation provides the imaging needed for the team to plan your treatments. This can be a lengthy, time-consuming process. Your team of radiation therapists, dosimetrists, physicists, and physicians must all play their roles in developing, approving, and quality assurance to be confident that everything looks good and that any errors or issues are found and resolved before you begin treatment on your first day.

For a great video explaining CT simulation visually, scan the QR code to watch "What to Expect: Radiation Therapy Simulation Appointment," which is on YouTube.com authored by Alliance Cancer Care on May 22, 2021.

CHAPTER 10
CT Simulation of the Brain or Skull

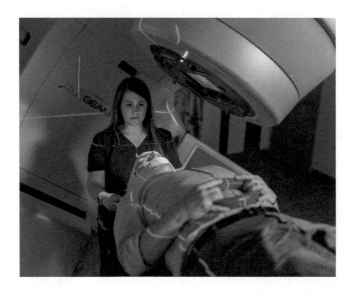

Figure 7 The radiation therapist places a customized thermoplastic mask over the patient's head to immobilize the patient before beginning radiation treatment to the brain. Image courtesy of Red Fox Photography.

Patients preparing to undergo treatment to their brain or skull will not have to change their clothing. However, you will be asked to take off any earrings that you are wearing as well as any necklaces. Please let your physician know if you have earrings or facial piercings that cannot be removed! Metal near the treatment area can affect certain aspects of your treatment, so your physician needs to be aware before you are scanned.

Hearing aids must also be removed. You will be asked to take your hair out of a ponytail if applicable and remove any hair clips that you might be wearing. It is preferable that you do not wear thick braids or have a wig on for treatment, so you might be asked to take those off. Removing any extra accessories on your head will help your treatment team reproduce your exact position each day by allowing your head to lay the same way each day. Also, if you have a thick beard and think you might want to shave it soon, do it BEFORE your simulation because shaving it afterward can greatly affect the way your mask fits for treatment.

Something as simple as shaving your beard off can have a great effect when it comes to your treatment position. Our work is very precise, down to sub-millimeters when possible. Shaving your beard or wearing a wig one day and not the next can alter the way your mask fits and therefore alter its ability to keep your head in the same position for treatment. The goal of simulating your treatment position is to be able to reproduce that very same setup each day. We want everything to be as close as possible to the original position every day that you receive treatment. This is vital to ensure that you are receiving the correct dose of radiation to the correct area of your brain/skull. In between treatments, you can put these back on. However, you should not wear them during the treatment to enable the team to deliver the most precise treatment possible.

The patient will be lying flat on the table. The table will have some type of frame on it that might look like a person's body or head outline. On the frame will be a headrest to go under your neck and offer support as well as help to tilt your head into a certain position. There are a variety of different headrests that help to tilt the head to different angles depending on what your physician recommends.

There will also be some type of cushion under your knees to make you more comfortable and relieve a little pressure off your back. You might be asked to either have your arms by your sides or to keep your hands on your abdomen or pelvis. You might be holding a ring, clasping your hands together, or holding a towel from either end. Whichever your medical team decides, they will let you know. It is important to note that every other body part is being kept down and away from the area of treatment.

Finally, a warm and wet mask will be placed over your face to conform to the shape of your head. It will be clipped into the board that you are lying on, immobilizing your head from just below your chin to the top of your head.

The last step of making your mask is the most important. The mask is made of a thermoplastic material that has holes throughout it so you can breathe with the mask on. As time passes, the material will cool and harden. It begins as a hard and flat object. It is put into either a hot water bath or into an "oven" and will begin to soften over the course of a couple of minutes. This makes it pliable so that it can be stretched and made to conform to the shape of your head and facial structures. This allows the team to outline your nose, chin, and top of your head. The better conformed your mask is, the better the likelihood that it holds you in the perfect position each day for treatment.

If you are claustrophobic, let your team know! Try to remind yourself that there are little holes all over the mask that you will be able to breathe through. If your anxiety and claustrophobia are severe, you may need to consult with your physician about the possibility or necessity of daily anxiety medication to help get you through your treatments. For patients in these cases, please be sure to have someone with you each day to drive you to and from your appointments.

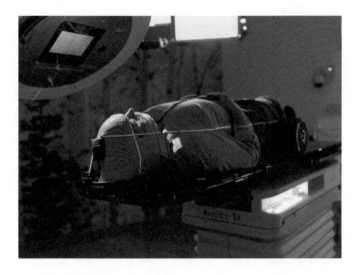

Figure 8 This patient is set up and in position to receive his radiation treatment to the brain. Image courtesy of Red Fox Photography.

According to the American Cancer Society, common short-term side effects resulting from radiation to the brain include the following:

1. Fatigue
2. Nausea and vomiting
3. Hair loss
4. Headaches
5. Skin and scalp changes
6. Cognitive changes
7. Seizures
8. Hearing loss

Please speak to your radiation oncologist and nurse about the potential side effects of your treatment to learn how to manage them. A couple of great additional resources to learn more about radiation to the brain can be found on YouTube. Scan these QR codes:

1. Radiation Oncology for Primary Brain Tumors – What You Need to Know (Interview with Dr. Lawrence Kleinberg) Authored by Johns Hopkins Medicine on January 17, 2017.

2. Radiation Therapy for Brain Tumors Video authored by ASTRO (American Society for Radiation Oncology) on July 12, 2017.

CHAPTER 11

CT Simulation & Treatment of the Head and Neck Region

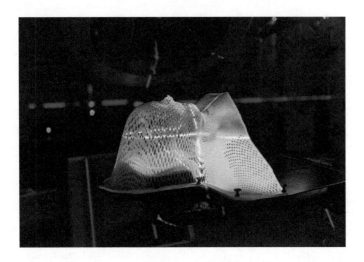

Figure 9 This image depicts a customized thermoplastic mask that is used to immobilize patients receiving radiation treatments to the head or neck areas. Image courtesy of Red Fox Photography.

H ead and neck treatment areas essentially cover anywhere from the top of the head down to the supraclavicular region (minus the brain, skull, and possibly c-spine). The setup and simulation position for a head and neck treatment area will be very similar to that of the brain treatment site. The major difference will be that the mask made for these patients will be longer and cover the top of the head down past the shoulders. The reason for this extra support is to consider the mobility of the shoulders, head, and neck. Ensuring that your shoulders are in the same exact position each day is essential, especially when the lymph nodes in your neck are being considered for treatment. Even if this is not the case for you, your physician might feel that immobilizing your shoulders will help create a more reproducible setup each day.

The head and neck masks will be made the same way as the shorter brain masks described in the brain section in the previous chapter. They, too, will clip into the frame you are laying on. Depending on the treatment area, your chin may be extended, tucked, or neutral.

Keep in mind that the mask will still have little holes so that you can breathe. Your physician might request that a mouthpiece, tongue depressor, or bite block be necessary for your treatment. Mouthpieces, tongue depressors, and bite blocks are very helpful in head and neck treatments. They can aid the team in keeping your tongue out of the treatment field or help bring your chin out of the treatment area.

Suppose we are treating a region of the mouth. In that case, these devices can also help ensure that this area is in the same position each day, resulting in an accurate and effective treatment, reducing radiation to areas that do not require treatment. Sometimes we will use bits of pink wax over a patient's teeth in areas where the bite blocks cause gum irritation.

Your physician will determine any additional aids used in treatment. If you have any questions about why something is necessary, ask!

Please also be sure to let your team know if you are wearing dentures. Sometimes you will be asked to remove them for treatment, and your team will need to take note of this in your chart. As for the brain setup, the same goes for the rule on hairstyles. If you are wearing a wig, it may need to be removed to help with setup reproducibility from day to day. If you have braids in on your simulation day, it's especially important to keep them in and wear them the same way each day for the duration of your treatment. Changing your hairstyle can result in difficulty setting you up, and you may need to be re-simulated later.

The same rules for jewelry apply to this treatment area as it did for the brain. You will be asked to remove all jewelry in the head and neck region. This applies to necklaces, earrings, nose rings, hair clips, brow piercings, etc. Let your team know if you have any piercings that cannot be removed, as this may affect the way your treatment is planned. Hearing aids will also need to be removed.

Another thing to note is that patients with facial hair must do their best to maintain the style they wore on their simulation day. It seems like a small thing, but we work in millimeters. If you had a nice full beard on your first day for simulation but then decide two weeks in that you want to shave it...you will not set up the same each day for treatment. The mask will be loose. You do have some control over how perfectly you set up for treatment. Please hold up your end of the treatment deal and stick to the same hairstyle/facial hairstyle you promised to keep on that first day. It only benefits YOU and your treatment. You can do whatever you want with it when treatment is over.

One final note about head and neck simulations is that you will likely be asked to change into a gown. You will be asked to take off everything from the waist up. There are a couple of reasons for this. One reason is that extra clothing will make the mask tighter each day. Removing the clothing helps to control the variable of different thicknesses of clothing, making the mask fit differently each day and possibly decreasing the accuracy of your treatment. Another reason is that some clinics still tattoo a lot, so you might get a couple of tattoos at your simulation to help with daily positioning. You'll need to wear a gown so the tattoos can be visible each day. Additionally, if your clothing covers the treatment area, your clothing could create a "bolus effect" and increase the skin dose you receive.

Bolus effect defined: causes the dose that the skin receives to be higher, creating a higher potential for side effects regarding the skin, including irritation and sunburn effect.

According to the American Cancer Society (i), common short-term side effects resulting from radiation to the head and neck regions include:

1. Sore throat
2. Dry mouth
3. Open sores in the throat or mouth
4. Difficulty swallowing
5. Changes in taste
6. Nausea
7. Earaches
8. Tooth decay
9. Hair loss
10. Changes in skin texture
11. Stiffening of the jaw
12. Skin irritations much like a sunburn can happen if the neck area is being treated.

Please speak to your radiation oncologist and nurse about the potential side effects of your treatment to learn how to manage them. A great additional resource to learn more about radiation to the head and neck region can be found on YouTube. Scan this QR code:

"Radiation Therapy for Head and Neck Cancers Video," authored by ASTRO on July 12, 2017.

CHAPTER 12
CT Simulation & Treatment of the Breast(s)

B reast treatments are one of the most common radiation treatments delivered to women. While breast cancer can most certainly occur in men, it is most common in females. Unfortunately, this is an extremely sensitive area of the body and can leave the patient vulnerable and exposed. This may not make you feel any better, but we are professionals and will do our best to help you maintain some sense of modesty.

Women are often agitated after their simulation because they don't expect us to be as "touchy" as we are. I hate to be the bearer of bad news, but this is one of the most awkward and touchy/hands-on setups we must perform, so we understand when our patients feel embarrassed. I truly do apologize, but unfortunately, this is the way treatment must be conducted.

The breast is one of our more difficult treatment areas because breast tissue is so movable, the breasts are close to the heart, skin folds in the axillary area, and breasts can vary significantly in size from patient to patient. We must ensure that the breast is positioned in a way that makes sense for what the physician hopes to achieve. Your physician will likely decide the best position based on all they have seen in their experience. There are a few most common setups for breast patients, but the immobilization devices and techniques used may differ from location to location.

Supine

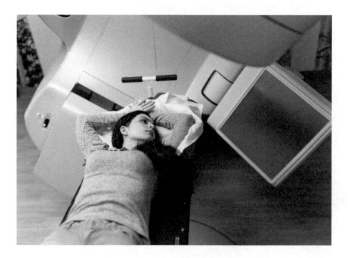

Figure 10 A patient expecting radiation treatment to the breast is in her setup position. Image courtesy of Red Fox Photography.

A patient lying in the supine position would mean the patient is lying on their back. The patient will be lying on some breast board with their arms up above their head. There might be a slight incline. This can be difficult for some patients if they have had surgery on the breast or axillary area. Since your arms will be up, please let your team know if you are experiencing any pain at the time of your simulation. This is very important! Your simulation appointment will be quick, but some of your treatment days will be longer! Suppose you are in extreme discomfort on your simulation day, and your physician's team plans your treatment based on your position. Any adjustments will likely only be possible by starting the process all over again. If you openly communicate with the team from the beginning, it will save time and effort on everyone's behalf. You also want to tell them if you're experiencing any discomfort because if you are experiencing it in the first session, it is likely that you will feel it going forward in your treatment as well. We want you to be as comfortable as possible while receiving your treatment!

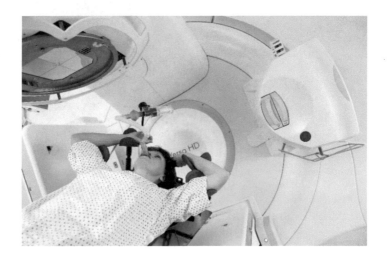

Figure 11 A patient is set up using the Active Breathing Coordinator device for breath-hold technique. Image(s) courtesy of Elekta.

When being treated lying supine, your physician might ask that you be simulated and treated using a breath-hold technique. This technique varies from organization to organization, but some sites can track your breathing and allow treatment to happen when you inhale. This technique is generally called the deep inspiration breath hold technique. The way this technique works is you will be instructed to take a deep breath in and then hold your breath. Treatment will only occur while you are in that breath-hold. This might be because the area of the breast(s) that requires treatment may be close to the heart. Taking a deep breath will cause your lungs to expand and your diaphragm to pull your heart away from your chest. This helps to decrease the radiation dose being delivered to your heart. Radiation dose to the heart is a big concern, especially for patients being treated to the left breast since your left breast is closer to your heart. Dose to the heart might lead the patient to a greater risk for coronary heart disease. (https://my.clevelandclinic.org/) Make sure to talk to your physician if you are at risk for heart disease.

Prone Position

Another technique for treating breast cancer patients is to treat the patient lying *face down* or what we call the "prone" position. The patient will be lying on a prone breast board. The patient's arms will be extended above the head, and hands will hold pegs. The unaffected breast will remain on top of the board, while the breast of interest will hang down over the side. This allows treatment to be delivered only to the affected breast. Often, we see this technique utilized for women with larger breasts or in cases where the dose to the heart is an increased concern or where the tumor bed is centrally located in the breast.

For all breast treatment setups, you will almost certainly be asked to change into a gown. Be prepared to remove all clothing from the waist up, including your bra. The point of the simulation is to get you into a reproducible setup position. So, the gown will help eliminate changes in clothing thickness and make the treatment area more accessible. Also, sometimes, the bra has metallic components, and we do not want metal in the treatment field where possible. In any case, different bras hold breast shapes differently, so to minimize changes from day to day, we ask you to remove them from the picture.

While your team is made up of medical professionals, some female patients can become very anxious about having males in the room because of religious reasons or to preserve modesty. This is entirely understandable! You can and should ask if having only females on the team is an option. This is YOUR journey! However, sometimes having a male present may have to occur, depending on staffing composition or the physical capability of the patient. Talk to your physician during your consultation to find out if it is possible only to have females present for your treatment.

If a clinic only has a couple of therapists and they are primarily men, you might need to choose a treatment time that would ensure the female therapists can be present for your treatment each day. Let your team know your preference so you won't be uncomfortable on your first day of treatment. This will help your treatment team plan and be better prepared to accommodate your request. Remember, there is no guarantee the team can accommodate your request, but we will try our best!

Lateral Decubitus

Lying in the lateral decubitus position essentially means lying *on your side*. If you are being treated for your left breast, you will be lying on your right side. The opposite goes if you are being treated for your right breast. You might have a cushion between your knees and a pillow under your head, with your arm under your pillow to support your head. This treatment position is typically utilized for patients receiving "boosts" to their original treatment site.

Electron Boost

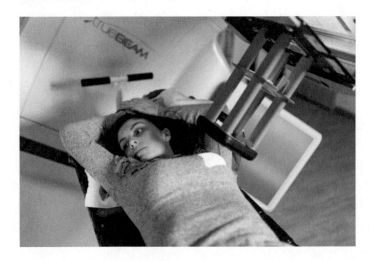

Figure 12 A patient is set up for an electron boost treatment to the left breast. Image courtesy of Red Fox Photography.

57

Patients undergoing radiation therapy treatments to the breast may require a "boost." Sometimes, the boost is to achieve scar sterilization, to kill any possible traces of cells in the scar area due to surgery. It may also be needed to achieve the doses necessary to reach optimal treatment goals. Neither you nor your treatment team may know immediately if your physician plans to add more boost treatments to your treatment plan. As your treatment course progresses, your physician will make their decision and will let you and your therapists know if it will be necessary.

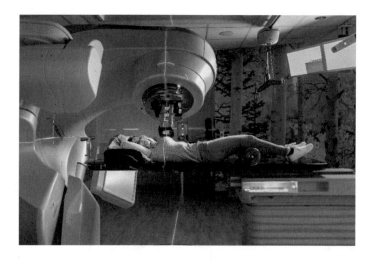

Figure 13 A side view of the setup position for a patient receiving an electron boost treatment to the left breast. Image courtesy of Red Fox Photography.

According to the American Cancer Society, (i) common short-term side effects resulting from radiation to the breast include:

1. Skin irritation
2. Skin dryness or change in color
3. Soreness of the breast
4. Lymphedema

Please speak to your radiation oncologist and nurse about the potential side effects of your treatment and learn how to manage them. YouTube is a great additional resource for learning more about radiation to the breast(s). Scan the following QR codes:

1. "Radiation Therapy to Treat Breast Cancer: Options, Duration, and Side Effects" authored by Yerbba-Breast Cancer on September 18, 2020.

2. "Radiation Therapy for Breast Cancer" authored by ASTRO on December 23, 2014.

3. "Active Breathing Device (ABC) Device for Breast Cancer" authored by Cleveland Clinic on May 6, 2021.

CHAPTER 13
CT Simulation and Treatment of the Thorax and Abdomen

(Liver, lung, pancreas, esophagus, T-spine, stomach)

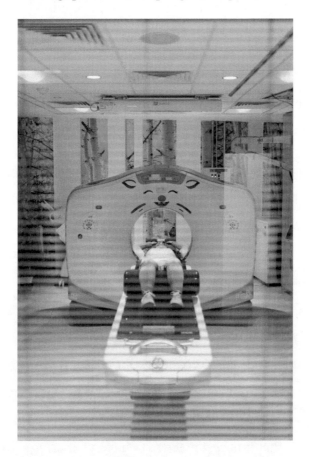

Figure 14 A patient is set up on the CT simulation table. Every patient is always in sight of a radiation therapist while their scan is being performed. Image courtesy of Red Fox Photography.

61

atients who are going to be simulated for treatments to the chest and abdominal areas will likely be expected to change into a gown and remove all their clothing from the waist up. Typically, we will place tattoos or skin markings with stickers on your chest and abdomen to help get you into position each day. These marks will help us to line you up quickly. Patients treated in these areas may or may not need the breath-hold technology. Please see the breast section on the deep inspiration breath hold technique.

Positioning

A few different ways you might be positioned for treatment to the chest and abdominal areas might be as follows:

- Headrest on top of a "wing board" with your arms extended above your head, holding onto pegs and your elbows winged out. With or without the breath hold technology, a knee cushion will be under your knees for comfort. This position is shown in *Figure 14*.

- Body mold cushion under your upper body and abdomen. Your arms will be above your head, holding pegs or a ring with a knee cushion under your knees. If you do not have great arm or shoulder mobility, your physician might plan your treatment with your arms down at your sides. Please note that it is best practice to have your arms above your head when possible so that we can prevent delivering doses to the arms. As always, we will leave this critical decision to your physician to make the best choice for you, but always speak up if you are experiencing any pain from the position that you are in.

- If you are receiving palliative radiation treatments to the spine, you might be positioned flat on your back with a headrest under your head. You might have a knee cushion under your knees for comfort with your arms at your sides.

Patients receiving radiation treatments to target the liver might be planned with an abdominal compression paddle. This device is often used with patients who are not candidates for the breath hold technique. The compression paddle helps decrease the motion in the abdominal area. It could be uncomfortable, so always let your treatment team know if it is causing any pain.

With these types of treatments, your physician might give you specific food and drink instructions to follow for the duration of your treatments. Your doctor might give you NPO orders, meaning no food or drink for a specific time before treatment. Please follow these instructions! It helps us control the variability of the treatment area daily. If you ever forget to follow the instructions, please let your treatment team know so they can ask the physician to look closely at your X-rays to decide if you can receive treatment that day.

Having your arms above your head can become difficult for someone with shoulder mobility issues. Suppose you find that your position is becoming too painful for you to maintain. In that case, consider taking Tylenol or some other type of pain medication before treatment to help you tolerate treatment a little better. Please *speak to your physician* if this is a concern of yours.

According to the American Cancer Society, (i) common short-term side effects resulting from radiation to the chest include:

1. Loss of appetite
2. Sore throat
3. Swallowing problems
4. Cough
5. Shortness of breath

According to the American Cancer Society, (i) common short-term side effects resulting from radiation to the abdomen include:

1. Nausea
2. Stomach cramps
3. Vomiting
4. Constipation
5. Diarrhea

Please speak to your radiation oncologist and nurse about the potential side effects of your treatment to learn how to manage them. A few great additional resources to learn more about radiation to the chest or abdomen can be found on YouTube. Scan these QR codes:

1. "Meicen SBRT Immobilization & Positioning System Instructional Video" authored by Meicen Med on December 2, 2020.

2. "Active Breathing Coordinator (ABC) Device for Lung Cancer or Abdominal Tumors" authored by Cleveland Clinic on October 31, 2019.

3. "Radiation Therapy for Lung Cancer" authored by ASTRO on December 23, 2014.

CHAPTER 14
CT Simulation and Treatment of the Pelvis, Supine

(Prostate, female GYN, pelvic nodes, lumbar/sacral spine)

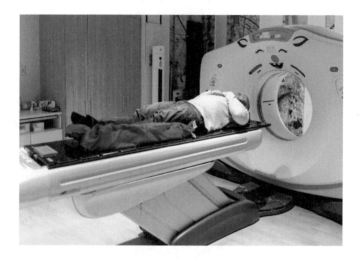

Figure 15 A patient is set up on the CT simulation table in a common treatment position for a patient receiving treatment to the pelvis. Image courtesy of Red Fox Photography.

Patients receiving treatment in the pelvic area will be treated very similarly. They will lie on a carbon fiber table with some type of headrest under their heads. They might have a cushion under their knees or an immobilization device, keeping the feet or legs still.

They may hold a blue ring on their chest to keep their arms in the same position or be instructed to clasp their hands together on their chest. If a patient is unable to hold their arms up on their own, the therapy team can offer some support by placing a strap around the arms and around the table to keep the patient's arms and hands up and out of the treatment area.

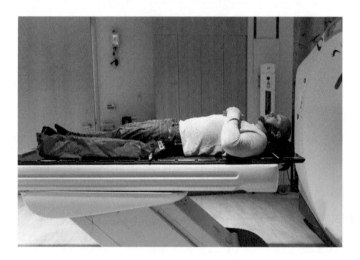

Figure 16 Side view of Figure 15. A patient is set up in a treatment position on the CT simulator. Image courtesy of Red Fox Photography.

We will do our best to help you maintain modesty as we set you up. We will place marks or tattoos on your hips, sides, or abdomen. Sometimes, the female patients will be positioned with their legs frog-legged. This means we will have you lying down, cushion under your head, with your bottom in a vacuum-sealed bag, your knees pointing outward in each direction, and your feet close together. This is a very awkward position for patients, and they might feel very vulnerable. Again, we do our best to maintain patients' modesty and will keep you covered as best as possible. This position is crucial because it can help us decrease the dose to other areas in the thighs, pelvic, and genital regions while still treating the exact areas to which we intend to deliver a specific dose.

Patients being simulated for treatment to the prostate or surrounding regions might be asked to arrive with a full bladder and achieve an empty rectum for their daily treatment. These are difficult things to ask and do. However, they are essential tasks. A full bladder helps push your bowel out of the treatment field. The reason why this is so important is because it will help to decrease the gastrointestinal (GI) side effects that you might experience throughout your treatments. Reducing the size of your rectum minimizes the dose to the rectum. Maintaining a full bladder and empty rectum together can help to keep the prostate in the same position each day, maximizing consistency in positioning from day to day.

If your bladder is consistently empty and you receive treatment, you increase your chances of experiencing diarrhea, upset stomach, nausea, vomiting, and stomach cramps. You probably do not wish to experience these things, so try to stay hydrated and fill your bladder for treatment. While your physician will have the best advice for you to achieve this, I offer my best tip: sip on water throughout the day! This will help you stay hydrated so that when you are trying to fill your bladder, the extra water can make it to your bladder rather than hydrating the dehydrated cells in your body.

Another thing that may be asked of a patient being treated for the prostate is that they come to treatment with an empty rectum. This, again, is a difficult thing to ask someone to do. It sounds so easy to tell someone to try to have a bowel movement each day, but it can be a rather challenging task for people who are not "regular" with their bowel movements. Please ask your physician or nurse for advice on attaining a full bladder and an empty rectum for treatment. They might offer you a list of food items to avoid and can recommend foods/medications to help you have a bowel movement if you struggle to have one.

CHAPTER 15
CT Simulation and Treatment of the Pelvis, Prone

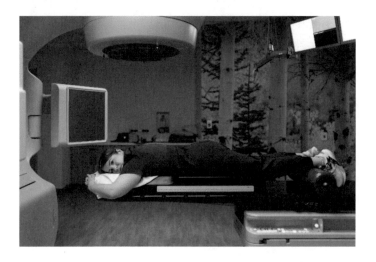

Figure 17 The radiation therapist is simulating the setup position for a prone treatment to the pelvis. Image courtesy of Red Fox Photography.

Sometimes, the physician will treat a patient with the patient lying on their stomach or in the "prone" position. You can discuss this with your physician as to their reasoning for the positioning preference. Often, this is the best way to treat tumors that are protruding from the anus because there is better access to the area of concern this way. The patient, in this case, would be lying on their stomach on a "belly board" where their stomach is hanging into a cut out on the board. This helps move the

70

abdomen and bowel away from the area we are trying to treat. You can relax with your head down like you would on a massage table, with your face inserted into a little cushion and arms up around the top of the board.

According to the American Cancer Society, (i) common short-term side effects resulting from radiation to the pelvis (bladder, ovarian, prostate) include:

1) Bladder issues such as
   - Pain or burning sensation when urinating
   - Difficulty urinating
   - Blood in the urine
   - Increased frequency of urination
2) Fertility issues
3) Nausea or vomiting
4) Constipation
5) Diarrhea

Please speak to your radiation oncologist and nurse about the potential side effects of your treatment to learn how to manage them. A few great additional resources to learn more about radiation to the male or female pelvis can be found on YouTube. Scan the following QR codes:

1. "Radiation Therapy for Gynecologic Cancers Video" authored by ASTRO on July 12, 2017.

2. "Treating Prostate Cancer with Radiation Therapy- Dr. Daniel Song" authored by Hopkins Kimmel on July 29, 2020.

CHAPTER 16
CT Simulation and Treatment of Extremities

(Shoulder, leg, arm, hand, foot)

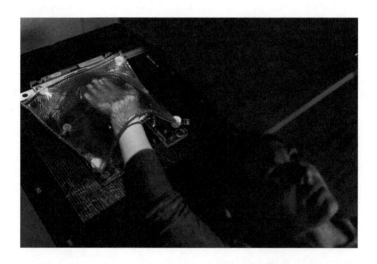

Figure 18 A patient is set up for treatment to the palm. 1 CM of bolus lays on top of the hand. Image courtesy of Red Fox Photography.

P atients being treated for an extremity might be experiencing pain. Speak to your physician about pain medication if you need help controlling pain levels. If your physician agrees that you will not be able to hold still long enough to complete your treatment each day, please consider taking pain medication like Tylenol to help you tolerate treatment a little better.

Treatment positioning for extremities can vary widely. It's almost like an anything-goes situation, where we will try everything to help us get your body part into a position that will allow the treatment machine to treat that area without putting you in danger of getting hit by the machine. It truly depends on the clinic you go to and the techniques it has found to work well.

A patient receiving treatment to the back of the arm could be asked to stand beside the treatment table with their palm facing down, gripping the edge of the far end of the table. That might be their treatment position. Someone else might be treated lying down on their stomach with their arm extended above their head.

A patient receiving radiation to the foot might be treated similarly to a pelvis patient, with a cushion under the head and a cushion molded around the legs. Someone else might have a mask molded around their foot, as it would be for a brain or head/neck setup.

A patient receiving treatment to the thigh or lower leg will be treated similarly to how a person being treated to the pelvis might be. A cushion under the head with a large mold made around the legs, with the affected leg straight and the unaffected leg "frogged" out.

A patient receiving treatment for the shoulder or other parts of the arm might be lying on a wing board like a patient being treated for the chest or abdomen, but their arms are down to their side, and the affected arm is winged out instead of above their head.

Extremities can be some of the most difficult or most straightforward positions for therapists to set up. Because extremities contain different joints and moveable parts surrounding them, we rely heavily on skin markings to help get you into position each day. If your therapists use a marker to make setup markings on your skin and put a bunch of stickers on you, they might beg you not to lose those stickers. Setting up these body parts can be very difficult and time-consuming. Those stickers help speed up the setup process for themselves and decrease the time you are in a potentially uncomfortable position.

CHAPTER 17
CT Simulation and Treatment: Total Body Irradiation

Total body irradiation, or TBI, is a technique that can be utilized as part of a pre-transplant conditioning regimen for patients about to undergo a stem cell or bone marrow transplant. These patients are often being treated for leukemia, a cancer of the blood-forming tissues. However, TBI has also been used to treat other diseases. As the name of this type of treatment indicates, TBI distributes radiation to all parts of your body. This can help to suppress the patient's immune system and increase the chances of the transplant being successful by decreasing the risk of the person's body rejecting the transplanted tissue.

With this type of treatment, different hospitals and clinics will have their techniques for setup and treatment. However, the goal for each location will be to get you into a position where treating your entire body with the same dose at the same time is possible. A bolus material may be placed on the patient's neck to act as a tissue compensator since the neck is often thinner than the rest of the body. A therapist might place a spoiler in front of the bed. The spoiler helps to ensure that an even dose is delivered to the patient's entire body. Different types of shielding may be used for the lungs or testicles. This is something your physician will consider if necessary for your treatment.

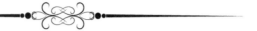

CHAPTER 18
Re-Simulation

S ometimes, a patient must repeat the CT simulation process. There could be multiple reasons why a patient might need to undergo the simulation process more than once throughout their radiation therapy journey. Some patients experience side effects that cause them to lose significant weight. Because the goal of the simulation is for a treatment plan to be developed based on the position you were in for the simulation, any substantial changes in weight, body size, body shape, or physical ability and mobility can make a significant impact on how you set up each day for treatment. Therefore, if any of these occur, you might need to undergo the process again. Please know there is nothing wrong about repeating this process. It happens occasionally, and the team needs to ensure proper treatment in the correct locations.

CHAPTER 19
Linear Accelerators and the Treatment Room

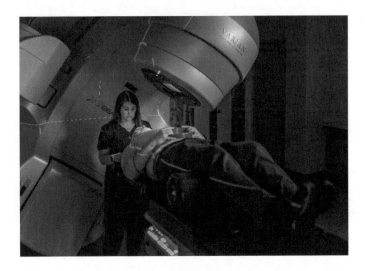

Figure 19 The radiation therapist is in the treatment room setting up a patient for radiation therapy treatment on the linear accelerator. Image courtesy of Red Fox Photography.

While every radiation oncology department will look different, the machines usually look similar. As with any other large machine or piece of equipment, there are significant brands that you will find in any given department. The brands, Varian and Elekta are the two frontrunners of linear accelerator technology.

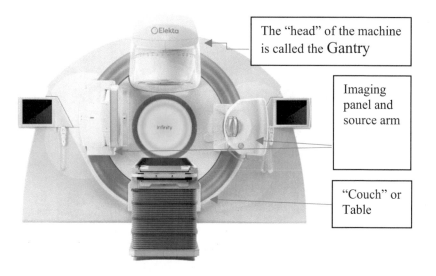

The "head" of the machine is called the Gantry

Imaging panel and source arm

"Couch" or Table

Figure 20 Elekta Infinity Linear Accelerator. Image(s) courtesy of Elekta.

The different MAJOR parts of the machines and their purposes include the following:

Gantry: This is where the radiation is being delivered from. This part of the machine (along with the others) will rotate around you but will not touch you.

Treatment Couch: This is the carbon fiber table on which you will lie for daily treatment. The tabletop can be moved to allow the therapists to maneuver you into the correct position. It can be raised or lowered, shifted laterally to either side and moved in and out longitudinally. Some treatment machines have the capability to adjust the table by pitch, roll, and yaw.

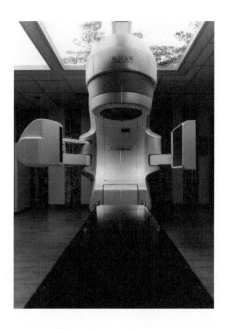

*Figure 21 Varian TrueBeam linear accelerator. Image
courtesy of Red Fox Photography.*

Imaging panels and source arm: The physician's
preference and hospital policy will determine the type of imaging
conducted before your treatment each day. The KV panel and
source arm allow therapists to take mini-CT scans to ensure you
are lying in the correct position before being treated. This helps
to deliver radiation to the treatment area with high accuracy.
Your therapists can also take x-rays from different angles (0, 90,
180, and 270 degrees) to ensure that you are laying in the correct
position.

A great educational video on how a linear accelerator
works can be found on Elekta's YouTube channel. Scan the QR

code: "How a Linear Accelerator Works- Elekta", authored by Elekta on December 26, 2010.

Other Treatment Machines

While the images shared above are the most common types of machines you'll see being used in traditional radiation oncology departments in the United States, there are many others that you might see. These are very specialized equipment, and you might have to research where the closest clinic to you may be that has these machines. I'll briefly share some of them with you.

MR Linac

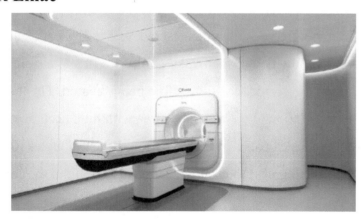

Figure 22 "MR-Linac" full room side view image. Image(s) courtesy of Elekta.

This is a linear accelerator that utilizes magnetic resonance imaging throughout the treatment. It decreases the dose being given off through imaging while increasing the accuracy and precision of the radiation through increased imaging during each treatment. Patients who want more information on this technology can find a link under Additional Resources.

Brachytherapy

Brachytherapy, or internal radiation therapy, is a local treatment that treats only a specific part of your body. With this type of treatment, a radiation source is placed in your body, which would then be placed in or near the tumor/tumor bed. It is often used to treat cancers of the head and neck, breast, cervix, prostate, and eye. For more resources, please see Additional Resources.

CyberKnife

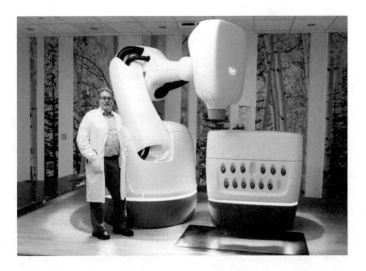

Figure 23 Medical Physicist standing next to the CyberKnife. Image courtesy of Red Fox Photography.

The CyberKnife System is a noninvasive treatment that can be used to treat areas throughout the body, including the brain, head and neck, spine, lung, prostate, lung, liver, pancreas, and kidney. It can be used as an alternative to surgery or for patients with inoperable or surgically complex tumors. Treatments are typically performed in one to five sessions. Please see Additional Resources for a link to learn more.

GammaKnife

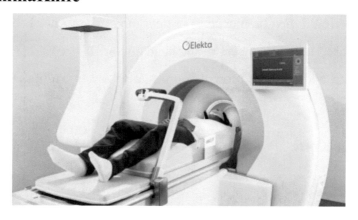

Figure 24 Patient in the treatment position for GammaKnife Radiosurgery. Image(s) courtesy of Elekta.

Gamma Knife radiosurgery, or stereotactic radiosurgery, is a type of radiotherapy treatment. Even though it's called surgery, a Gamma Knife procedure doesn't use incisions. It also isn't a knife. Gamma Knife uses very precise beams of gamma rays to treat an area of disease (lesion) or growth (tumor). It's most often used in the brain. The beams of gamma radiation send a very intense dose of radiation to a small area without making an incision. Radiosurgery destroys cells so they can't grow and will cause a lesion or tumor to shrink over time.

Gamma Knife radiosurgery is called surgery because the result is similar to removing a lesion with surgery. The radiation beams are precisely focused to reach the lesion, with little effect on nearby healthy tissue. (Johns Hopkins Medicine)

Proton Therapy

Proton therapy is a type of radiation therapy treatment that uses high-powered energy to treat cancer and some noncancerous tumors. Radiation therapy using X-rays has long been used to treat these conditions. Proton therapy is a newer radiation therapy that uses energy from positively charged particles (protons). Proton therapy has shown promise in treating several kinds of cancer. Studies have suggested that proton therapy may cause fewer side effects than traditional radiation since doctors can better control where the proton beams deliver their energy. However, few studies have compared proton and X-ray radiation, so it's unclear whether proton therapy is more effective at prolonging lives. Proton therapy isn't widely available, although new proton therapy centers are being built in the United States and other countries. (Mayo Clinic website)

CHAPTER 20
Radiation Is Prescribed

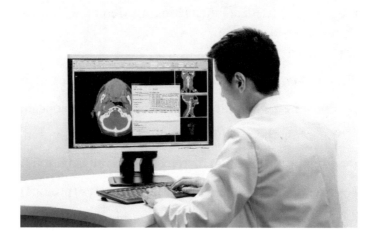

Figure 25 A treatment plan is in progress. Image(s) courtesy of Elekta.

Y ou may be thinking about your traditional prescriptions, where your doctor sends a note to the pharmacy, and you pick up the medication. It is similar, but radiation therapists administer the dose with the beams rather than picking up the medication, targeting the specific area needing treatment. Instead of milligrams, traditional radiation uses Grayscale to prescribe radiation doses. Your prescription may be read in Gray (Gy) or Centigray (cGy). Often, we see daily doses ranging from 180-200cGy per treatment for longer courses of treatment. Fewer treatments frequently indicate a higher daily dose of up to

1,000cGy. Everything all depends on the prescription determined and *prescribed* by your physician.

That said, it's important to address some questions that I have encountered as posed by patients throughout my career.

Commonly asked questions regarding radiation prescriptions:

Question: "Can we just double the treatment today so I can finish a day early?"

Answer: No, not if your prescription says treatment once a day. Your physician can change your prescription and authorize bi-daily treatment if they feel it is safe and reasonable. Still, it would never be a decision that your radiation therapists would make. Just like your nurse cannot make that decision in your family doctor's office, we cannot either. That decision is entirely up to the practicing physician.

Question: "Can I just come in on Tuesdays and Thursdays?"

Answer: If your prescription says treatment once daily for five days a week, then no. Treatments work best when you don't miss them! If prescribed once a day, you should receive treatments **every** day! Some patients will be treated fewer than five times a week, depending on the prescription your doctor orders. Different diagnoses might be best treated with treatments twice a week. Others are treated only once a week or every other day. Speak with your radiation oncologist to see what your treatment schedule is anticipated to be. *You can talk to your doctor about this to see if it is an option!*

Question: "Will I receive the same dose each day? "

Answer: Yes, the doctor and the treatment planning team create a treatment plan specific to each patient that your radiation therapists cannot deviate from. The physician and dosimetrist created your treatment plan with the goal of delivering a certain dose each treatment day. Sometimes, the doctor can give you a "day off" or change the plan. However, only the doctor can change that, not the therapist.

Question: "Am I getting better treatment if I get 20 treatments instead of 10 (Or ten instead of 20)?"

Answer: No, not necessarily. Treatment length is determined patient by patient, case by case, and diagnosis by diagnosis. Different body areas have different treatment protocols and standards of care regarding the best way to be treated. An immense amount of research backs these protocols and standards. Some patients receive five treatments, while others are prescribed 48. Many things go into the final decision for your treatment. Your doctor will have reviewed different options with you and given you their best recommendation based on years of experience, tons of knowledge, and accessible research.

Your physician wanted you to receive the dose the way they prescribed it for a reason. Your doctor is the expert in this field, and you must trust that they know what they are doing. If you are ever nervous or worried about something regarding your treatment, always ask questions if you need clarification. This is **YOUR** treatment. All questions are good if knowing the answers will help you feel more comfortable and better prepared to get through your treatments.

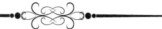

CHAPTER 21
On Treatment Visits and Tracking Progress

One way for the treatment team to stay updated on each patient's progress and how they are tolerating their treatments is by way of "on-treatment visits," or OTVs. These appointments are scheduled on your behalf to meet with your radiation oncology nurse and oncologist. These visits are the perfect time to ask your doctor any questions that you might have about your treatment progress and to mention any side effects you might be experiencing. Ask questions and give accurate information about how you are feeling because the more information your team has, the better they can care for you. Nothing is too small or irrelevant regarding your treatment and overall health!

While processes can vary from clinic to clinic, often, a nurse or medical technician will first speak with you in an exam room. They will get a set of vital signs and an updated weight measurement to enter into your records. This updated information will help your team gather insight into the effects of the treatment on your body. Although these can be helpful indicators, it is crucial to communicate with your team. Please let the nurse or physician know if you are experiencing a difficult time eating, sleeping more than usual, not being able to sleep at all, having weakness, etc., so that they know to keep a watchful eye on you. This lets them offer recommendations and medical advice on treating different side effects. As medical professionals, we have seen it all, so please do not hesitate or feel embarrassed! We are here to help you to the best of our abilities!

Depending on the frequency of your treatments, you may see the physician once or twice a week for the duration of your treatments. While these are scheduled visits, you are always welcome to speak to a nurse if you have issues or concerns regarding therapy on any given day. If you have a question that your therapists cannot answer, please let your radiation therapy team know if you need to speak with someone, and they can help facilitate it.

CHAPTER 22
Scheduling Daily Treatment Appointment Times

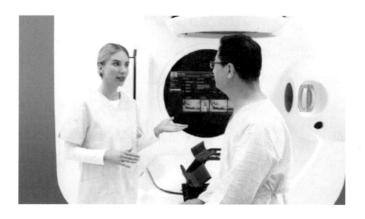

Figure 26 A female radiation therapist is speaking to the patient. Image(s) courtesy of Elekta.

Your treatment journey is going to be a hectic and likely inconvenient time of your life. You might have a lot of different appointments that you have to make it to, so finding a time that will work for you each day might seem overwhelming. We completely understand this and will always try our best to schedule you at times which are most convenient for you! Sometimes, we can be flexible depending on the clinic hours, how many treatments you will be getting, the duration of each treatment (10 minutes to an hour), and how busy the clinic is.

Unfortunately, there will also be times when we cannot be flexible with treatment times. It is sometimes challenging to squeeze an extra patient in if it is a hectic clinic and they are already treating patients back-to-back all day from 7 a.m. until 5 p.m. However, because we really want you to start your treatments and you truly do matter to us, we will offer the best times we can.

At this moment in time, you might feel like everything is out of your control. The time of your appointment might seem like another disappointment. Regardless of the time, it is essential to remember that *you are getting treatment.* And for this, you are so fortunate because there are so many people around the world who are not as lucky. Try to make the time work, even if it isn't your preferred time, because your health matters the most! Discuss this with your team if you cannot make the times work!

Many patients get very angry and yell at the therapists when they are frustrated. While we understand that you are frustrated about the times and not necessarily at us, please remember that we are all just doing our jobs to the best of our abilities. We wish we could accommodate every patient's ideal treatment time, but sometimes we simply cannot. At least, *not yet*! When one patient completes their treatment course, a time slot opens. If a time slot opens up during your treatment that might work better for you, we can always offer it to you when it

93

becomes available. Ask to get put on the waiting list for a specific timeframe.

As a practicing radiation therapist, I beg that you keep an open mind and be flexible. This is difficult, and it may seem like you are losing control or that we do not care. I promise that this is NOT typically the case! We will do our best to accommodate you and your schedule whenever possible!

If you genuinely think about it, virtually no medical centers out there can offer you any time you ask for. Radiation Therapy clinics are no different. While we value you as an individual and want to do everything we can to accommodate your requests, it would be unfair to ask another patient to change their time to give it to you. No patient is more important than another, so please don't ask us to value you more. However, we will work with you to find a time that is best for you if that is an option because you **<u>ARE</u>** important to us! Most of us went into this field because we have had family members or friends who fought cancer, moving us to join the fight. We care! I can promise that we indeed do!

CHAPTER 23
Arriving On Time and Prepared for Treatment

A lways arrive on time for your treatments! I mean this as respectfully as possible, but this is your *cancer* treatment. Does receiving your cancer treatment not mean enough to you to be on time for it? I certainly hope so! We understand that important things are happening in your life, and this is a hectic time. You have a million things going on, and we are not trying to minimize the struggle! However, many clinics have hectic schedules due to heavy patient volume. We respect each patient's time and do our best to take patients on time for their appointments. Remember that while we understand traffic and other obligations, being late impacts the schedule for all patients that follow your appointment. This makes us late for the next patient, the patient after that, the patient after that, and every patient for the rest of the day. You get it; it's a snowball effect. It is unfair to those other patients who were on time after you because, like you, they have other important things going on in their lives. You are not the only person receiving treatment that day, so please try your best to be on time for your appointment! It's the respectful thing to do.

While we fully expect you to be on time, changed, and **ready to enter the treatment room** at your given appointment time, we would love for you to arrive a little early. We completely understand that life can be hectic and that things happen. For this reason, most clinics will often ask patients to head to the clinic *early* with enough time to act as a buffer so traffic and other "unforeseeable" events have a lower impact on their ability to arrive on time.

Sometimes, even if you are on time or early, we might take you in late and ask you to be patient. Sometimes, this is due to the machine having a fault or error which we had to troubleshoot. Another patient might have been late. Another patient might not be feeling well, having difficulty with side effects related to their treatment, or be physically too weak to move quickly or require medical attention. Sometimes, patients need more of our time than we typically anticipate. We hope for grace and understanding in these situations because we strive to give each patient the care they deserve. This could be you one day, and we will always give you the extra time you need. **Please be patient and try to have a little grace for your fellow cancer warriors.**

Another reason the schedule runs late is that we sometimes need your physician's approval regarding your X-rays before we can treat you. Only physicians can approve these images, so we can only begin with that approval. Physicians have so many tasks that it may take a few minutes for us to get to them in their "queue." We will work as quickly and diligently as possible to get the approval and to get you started with your treatments each day.

So much work goes on behind the scenes once you have entered the treatment room. I promise we are not simply stepping out of the room and pushing a button. We are ensuring you are lined up correctly and we feel confident we will deliver the radiation to the correct location in your body. We do not want to rush this step because doing so could cause you adverse side effects and consequences, which you would like to avoid. Please trust that we are doing our best. I can guarantee that, as healthcare professionals, we also do not like running behind schedule. Sometimes, it might mean working through our lunch break or that we will not get off work on time. Trust me, after an emotionally draining day of caring for sick people, we have families that we would like to go home to as well. We understand the frustration, but please work with us to ensure your safety and the best care we can offer you.

CHAPTER 24
Radiation Oncology Team— It Takes a Village!

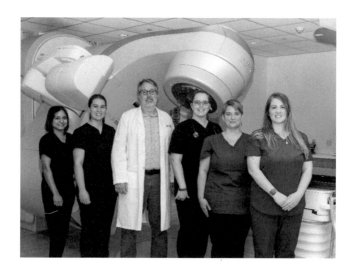

Figure 27 The radiation oncology team consists of a large group of people, some of whom you may never meet. Image courtesy of Red Fox Photography.

L ike any other healthcare department, radiation oncology is made up of many different groups of people focused on getting you the best possible treatment and care. Radiation oncology is comprised of administrative professionals, billing professionals, ancillary staff including cleaning professionals, patient transporters, IT workers, machine and software engineers, medical assistants, nurses, radiation therapists, dosimetrists, medical physicists, and, of course, physicians. Each profession is vital in making radiation oncology and your treatment run smoothly.

Medical assistants and oncology nurses: Supportive, caring, and knowledgeable medical staff who will provide medical care for you throughout your radiation journey.

Radiation therapists: Medical professionals trained to use the equipment that delivers your daily treatment. They will set you up for treatment each day. You will see your therapists more frequently than any other staff listed.

Medical dosimetrists: Professionals who create treatment plans using the orders and parameters given by the radiation oncologists. These are the behind-the-scenes staff who essentially design your treatment.

Medical physicists: These behind-the-scenes professionals ensure the quality and safety of the machines used for treatment. The physician and the physicist must approve every treatment plan.

Radiation oncologists: These medical doctors are responsible for your care throughout your treatment. They are the ones who decide on the best protocol to use for each treatment and what dose each patient should receive to accomplish the treatment goal effectively. They will prescribe your treatment in terms of dose per fraction, meaning how much radiation you should receive and for how many days you will receive it.

Mechanical/electrical engineers: Professionals specializing in repairing linear accelerators and other equipment used for daily radiation treatment.

IT: Information technology staff who help to keep computers, connectivity, and software working optimally.

Medical transporters and monitor technicians: Professionals transporting inpatients to and from their medical appointments. Patients are picked up in their hospital room and are transported by bed or wheelchair to the treatment room. If you expect to be admitted to the hospital for a planned procedure during your treatment course, please let a member of your radiation oncology staff team know. They will ensure that transport requests are entered daily to help facilitate your treatment while you are an inpatient.

Social workers are compassionate staff licensed to counsel people affected by cancer. They offer emotional support to patients, and, at some clinics, help set up transportation assistance and other practical things that prevent a patient from beginning or completing treatment.

Dieticians/nutritionists: Medically trained staff who work with oncology patients to develop a diet during radiation. They work with the patient to adjust their nutritional intake to minimize side effects caused by their treatments.

Front desk and administrative staff: These staff members perform various services. They oversee patient check-in, billing, scheduling, and more.

Commonly Asked Questions

Question: Am I radioactive? Can I be around my family?

Answer: We get this question very often! It is not a dumb question since it pertains to the safety of your family and friends! After receiving <u>traditional</u> radiation therapy, you are <u>not</u> radioactive. So, patients receiving external beam radiation therapy on a linear accelerator are not radioactive after their treatment. While the radiation does continue to work in your body at a cellular level, it cannot affect people around you. Try to repress the sci-fi movie scenes you have roaming around in your mind and feel safe knowing you can be around your family and friends without causing any harm! Take deep breaths and have the peace of mind of knowing that you cannot harm anyone around you by receiving your treatment!

Question: How much longer is the treatment going to take?

Answer: Patients or their loved ones can become aggressive with the therapist regarding how much longer they have left until they are done. I know you want us to push a magic button and cure you, but unfortunately, it is not that easy. We have many safety protocols, methods, and procedures in place to ensure that you are in the correct position and receiving the proper dose before we can start the radiation treatment. This is good for you because we ensure you receive the best possible treatment! Taking this time reduces radiation exposure to healthy tissue, allowing the treatment to be as concise as possible and better target unhealthy tissue. In the long run, this will help decrease any extra or unnecessary side effects you'll experience during and following your treatment.

Question: Can I record my treatment?

Answer: The quick and easy response to this question is that you cannot record your treatment. As with any business, there is a lot of red tape around photography in a hospital or clinic. The biggest reason is to ensure that no other patient's information is exposed to the public. Some clinics have a few extra minutes to allow you to bring a family member or friend into the treatment room if you want to show someone what you are experiencing each day.

Some clinics can take a photo of you on the treatment table so you can show your friends and family or keep it as a souvenir. Recording takes on a whole new life because anyone speaking must permit you to record them. Anyone visible must give you their permission to record them. Also, no patient information can be identified in your recording. Always ask for permission before taking photos or recording anything to prevent legal issues. Some facilities strictly prohibit taking photos.

If you want a photo or anything else like that, ask for permission because your team might be able to help accommodate parts of the request, as mentioned above.

Question: Can you see if the tumor is shrinking?

Answer: Unfortunately, even if we can see that the tumor is shrinking (or growing), we are not able to share that information with you. It is the physician's responsibility to share that type of information with a patient. The quality of the imaging we perform on a linear accelerator is not, however, of diagnostic quality. For that reason, you will be scheduled for a follow-up imaging scan after your treatments are complete. The physician will then be able to use those results to give you a more accurate answer to this question.

CHAPTER 25
Words of Encouragement

I know this is a tough time in your life and everything might seem overwhelming. Whether you are the person battling cancer yourself, are a family member who just found out the news, or are a friend bringing the patient to their treatment appointments, I know this is a challenging journey. There are so many emotions you might be feeling, possibly all at the same time: anger, fear, dread, hopelessness, sadness. Go ahead and feel those feelings! This does not make you weak or any other negative descriptor that is going through your mind! Hearing that you or a loved one has cancer is one of the scariest things you will ever hear. This is a vulnerable time, and your feelings are valid, regardless of what anyone else may expect or think!

I want to share with you, wherever you are on this journey, you are not in this alone! I hope you have a substantial home support system and clinical site. Everyone deserves to have someone in their corner, cheering them on and motivating them to continue. **You are worth it!** Your life and health are worth fighting for!

Unfortunately, many people may not have a friend or family member who can physically be there for treatment.

Whether that is because they live in another state or country, because their work will not provide the time off they need, or because they cannot afford to take the time off work—you are still not alone. Remember, you have your treatment team, and we will do our absolute best to support you on your journey.

Some clinics might be jam-packed. Unfortunately, they cannot always be your confidant and have an hour-long conversation about everything in your life, though they may try! We will be there with encouragement on days when you think you cannot keep going. We observe you daily to check for notable differences in weight loss, mood, or general well-being. We will ask you how your day is going, what your plans are for the weekend, and how you feel now.

While we are not mental health professionals, we can undoubtedly listen with an empathetic ear and offer our most sincere words of encouragement. Cancer treatment is not easy! We know this. But we will do our best to get you through your treatment course so that the radiation can do its job.

With all this being said, I genuinely want all of the support system members reading this book to understand what I am writing here. Cancer itself and cancer treatment are not a walk in the park. ***It's not easy***! Please do your best if you can physically be there for your loved ones during this process. This is not a battle anyone should fight on their own! If you cannot be there physically, try your best to be there emotionally. A few minutes of conversation, a few words of encouragement, checking in on them, telling them how much you love them and support them, sending a quick text, and anything else you can do to help them not feel alone will go a long way in helping their emotional state and their ability to keep fighting.

Treatment is a physical battle, yes. However, it is also quite a mental and emotional battle. I would not want to go through a cancer journey on my own, and I would certainly never let a friend or family member do it alone, either, if I had the chance. Showing them you are there as a member of their support system, physically present, or just as emotional support on the other end of a phone call could mean the world to them. Your support could get them through their most formidable challenge and hardest days when they are mentally exhausted.

Sometimes, it is just impossible for you to be there, which is entirely understandable. ***I am not here trying to shame you!*** This is tough for you, too! Life happens, and so many circumstances might make being present impossible. I ask that you try your hardest to be there when you can because your presence alone, emotionally or physically, could be just what your loved ones need to find the strength to keep fighting.

CHAPTER 26
Final Day of Treatment!

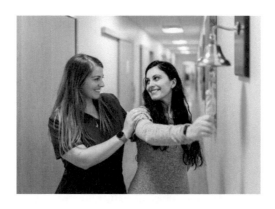

Figure 28 A patient rings the bell on her final day of treatment with the support of her radiation therapist. Image courtesy of Red Fox Photography.

Yay! You did it! You made it to the very last day of treatment and what a journey it has been! **<u>Congratulations</u>**! Your fight has been so courageous and inspiring to others and your team would love to celebrate this accomplishment with you. On your last day of treatment, you are welcome to bring family and friends to watch and celebrate with you as you ring the bell. Sometimes, patients who ring the bell are cancer-free, but this isn't always the case. Ringing the bell doesn't have to indicate this, but rather, show the world and yourself that you have accomplished yet another milestone in your fight against cancer.

While some centers may not have a bell for you to ring, I'm sure they each have a way to celebrate you on your last day, so be sure to ask the team. Congratulations, again, and good luck to you! Be sure to visit the team when you return for a follow-up to let everyone know how you're doing!

Index of Figures

Figure 3: Image(s) courtesy of Elekta. Agility-MultiLeaf-Shape.jpg (1500×1500) (elekta.com)

Figure 11: Image(s) courtesy of Elekta. Patient-Set-up-of-Active-Breating-Coordinator-on-Versa-HD.jpg (3042×1977) (elekta.com)

Figure 20: Image(s) courtesy of Elekta. Infinity-Linac-Front-on-View.png (2269×1859) (elekta.com)

Figure 22: Image(s) courtesy of Elekta. Elekta-Unity-Full-Room-Side-View-Image.jpg (1800×1799)

Figure 24: 'Image(s) courtesy of Elekta' elekta-esprit-patient-in-treatment-position-mask.jpg (2560×1707)

Figure 25, Image(s) courtesy of Elekta. Monaco-Treatment-Plan-in-Progress.jpg (2736×1824) (elekta.com)

Figure 28, Image(s) courtesy of Elekta. Female-RT-and-patient.jpg (6720×4480) (elekta.com)

Figures 1, 2, 4, 5, 6, 7, 8, 9, 10, 12, 13, 14, 15, 16, 17, 18, 19, 21, 23, 26, 27, and 29 are courtesy of Red Fox Photography.

Additional Resources

A video that does an incredible job introducing radiation therapy to the general public can be found on YouTube.com. Scan this QR code: "An Introduction to Radiation Therapy" authored by ASTRO (American Society for Radiation Oncology) on July 7, 2023.

You can utilize the following resources for additional information regarding cancer and radiation therapy:

1. American Cancer Society website
2. National Cancer Institute website
3. Mayo Clinic website
4. Most radiation oncology departments have their own website with information about their services. Perform a quick Google search!
5. To see a linear accelerator in action, look up "linear accelerator radiation therapy" on YouTube's search engine.

Other Treatment Machines

MR-Linac:
https://www.elekta.com/patients/mr-linac/

Ng J, Gregucci F, Pennell RT, Nagar H, Golden EB, Knisely JPS, Sanfilippo NJ, Formenti SC. MRI-LINAC: A transformative technology in radiation oncology. Front Oncol. 2023 Jan 27;13:1117874. doi: 10.3389/fonc.2023.1117874. PMID: 36776309; PMCID: PMC9911688.

Brachytherapy:
https://www.cancer.gov/about-cancer/treatment/types/radiation-therapy/brachytherapy

CyberKnife:
https://cyberknife.com/cyberknife-how-it-works/

GammaKnife:
https://www.hopkinsmedicine.org/health/treatment-tests-and-therapies/gamma-knife-radiosurgery#:~:text=Gamma%20Knife%20uses%20very%20precise,that%20they%20can't%20grow

Mayo Clinic:
https://www.mayoclinic.org/tests-procedures/brain-stereotactic-radiosurgery/about/pac-20384679

Proton Therapy:
https://www.mayoclinic.org/tests-procedures/proton-therapy/about/pac-20384758 (Mayo Clinic)

Endnotes

[i] **Radiation Therapy:**

Side Effects of Radiation Therapy | Radiation Effects on Body | American Cancer Society

External Beam Radiation | Types of External Radiation Therapy | American Cancer Society

[ii] **Heterotopic Bone Ossification**

Lee A, Maani EV, Amin NP. *Radiation Therapy for Heterotopic Ossification Prophylaxis*. [Updated 2022 Oct 3]. In: StatPearls [Internet]. Treasure Island (FL): StatPearls Publishing; 2024 Jan-. Available from: https://www.ncbi.nlm.nih.gov/books/NBK493155/

[iii] **Dupuytren's Contracture**

Kadhum M, Smock E, Khan A, Fleming A. Radiotherapy in Dupuytren's disease: a systematic review of the evidence. J Hand Surg Eur Vol. 2017 Sep;42(7):689-692. doi: 10.1177/1753193417695996. Epub 2017 Mar 13. PMID: 28490266. Available from: Radiotherapy in Dupuytren's disease: a systematic review of the evidence - PubMed (nih.gov)

[iv] **Superior Vena Cava Syndrome**.
Azizi, A, Shafi, I, Shah, N. et al. Superior Vena Cava Syndrome. J Am Coll Cardiol Intv. 2020 Dec, 13 (24) 2896-2910. https://doi.org/10.1016/j.jcin.2020.08.038

Made in the USA
Columbia, SC
02 March 2025